# Veggie-Wedgie Fruity-Tootie

## (A kid's guide to fruits and vegetables!)

By
Allison Ria Duran

# Acknowledgements

Written and conceived by Allison Duran
Layout and editing by Jonathan Duran

This book is dedicated to my family.
Gabriel, Simone, Jon and all the rest.

Let's teach kids to eat healthy and care about what they put into their bodies so that we may provide a better future for everyone.

# Introduction

The more I learned about food production in the US, the more passionate I became about healthy eating and sustainable living.

I have two children, and after watching friends and family members fight and lose their battles with diabetes and cancer, I knew it was time for a drastic change in our lives.

Luckily, I love to cook, so I have the daily opportunity to practice what I preach; out went the processed foods and hormone enhanced, pesticide soaked produce – then, in came organic, natural and farm fresh produce and ingredients. Our meals are now constantly filled with the foods covered in this book.

I'm dedicated to raising children that make wise choices when it comes to their health and their diet. I want them to be educated and have a genuine reason to objectively choose continuing on with this lifestyle choice when they finally grow up and leave home. At younger ages, it's all about the impression they get from the food in front of them; society has done a lot of damage and it's our job to attempt to reverse this. With this book I hope to show children that these foods are friendly, funny and that eating them can benefit them greatly!

I hope you enjoy reading this to your own children! Let's play with our food a bit, shall we?

# Veggie-Wedgie Fruity-Tootie

Green or red -
  I'm crunchy and absolutely delicious!

I am an **APPLE!!!**

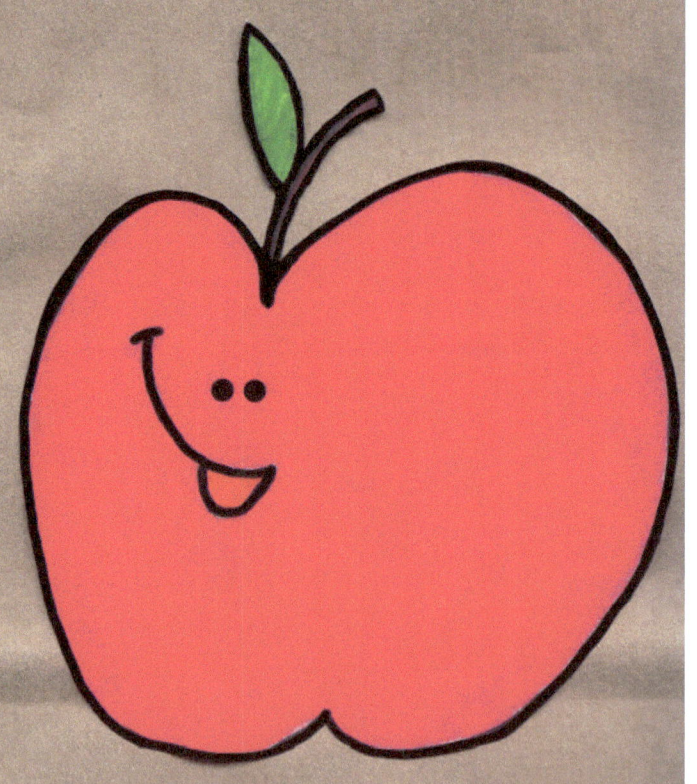

We Apples are pretty popular… and for good reason too; we protect your immune system and help to rid your liver of harmful toxins.

Eat me often and I will help you stay healthy! As the old saying goes: An apple a day keeps you healthy and paid… wait, that's not how it goes…

Yummy tip:

For a quick and simple treat, just slice and apple into wedges and serve with a peanut butter!

I'm an

# ARTICHOKE!!!

I'm as fun
to pronounce
as I am to eat!

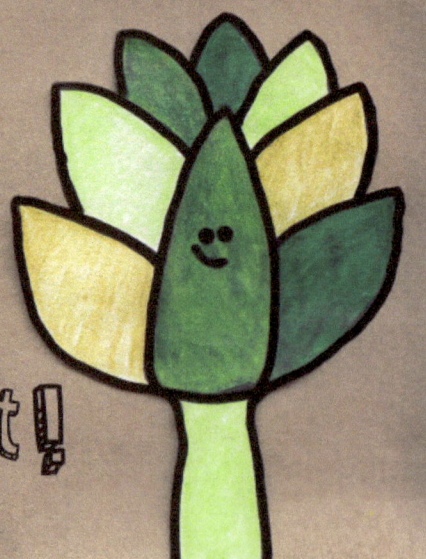

While I'm all about fun and games, I take my job as an artichoke very seriously!

Just like my good friends, Apples, I help your liver and keep it working at its best.

Livers are extremely important for processing your body's waste and a good strong liver is vital to a healthy life!

Yummy tip:
Steam a whole artichoke for 25-45 minutes (depending on size).Be sure to trim the leaves as they can be sharp!
Melt 4 TBSP of butter to use as a dipping sauce - or just use some olive oil containing a clove of garlic.

# A-vo-ca-do, that's me!

# I'm an AVOCADO!!!

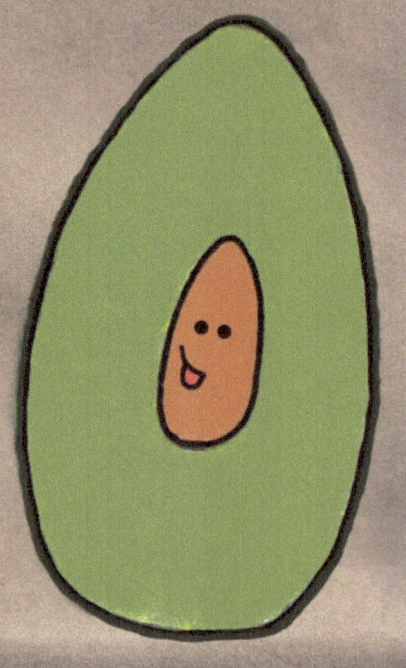

You know what? Being an avocado, I have a healthy kind of fat called monounsaturated fat – whew, that's a big word!

A big word that has big benefits! I can reduce the risk for diabetes and protect your heart.

Psssst… I also contain fiber that helps you poo! Woo!

Yummy tip:
Avocados are amazing on their own! Kids love them because of their mild taste and creamy texture. You can simply discard the pit, scoop out the avocado, and sprinkle with fresh lime juice and a pinch of salt.

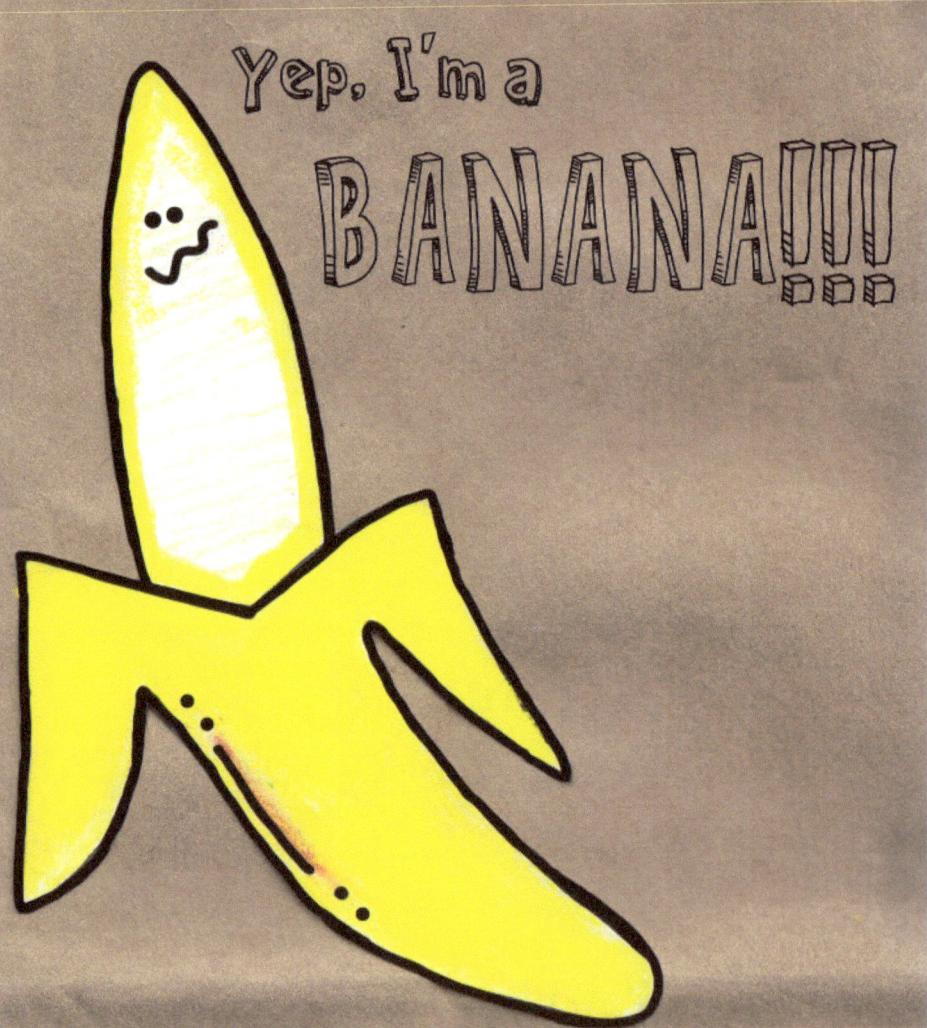

Since I'm a super-cool banana, I'm full of vitamin B-6, which helps to clean your blood and helps you feel relaxed!

Need a snack before bed? I'm a great choice!

Yummy tip:
Slice a ripe banana and freeze. Then, simply add it to your next smoothie of yogurt, milk, blueberries or whatever it is that you desire – bananas go great with all kinds of tastes!

I can be
red, green, yellow or orange!

I'm a...

BELL PEPPER!!!

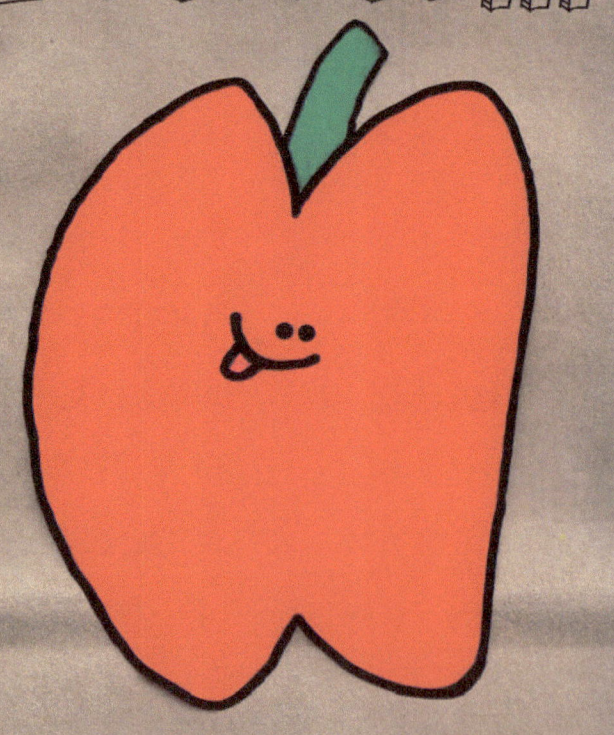

Bell peppers like me reduce your risk for heart disease and cancer. Heck, we can even help relieve symptoms of asthma!

I taste sweet and I'm wonderfully crunchy!!

Yummy tip:
Slice a fresh bell pepper into strips and sauté in a TBSP of olive oil. Then add some other veggies you may have lying around; mushrooms, onions, corn, etc. Cook this mixture 5-10 minutes or until done. Wrap the mix in a whole wheat tortilla and top with salsa, hummus or some of your favorite cheese!

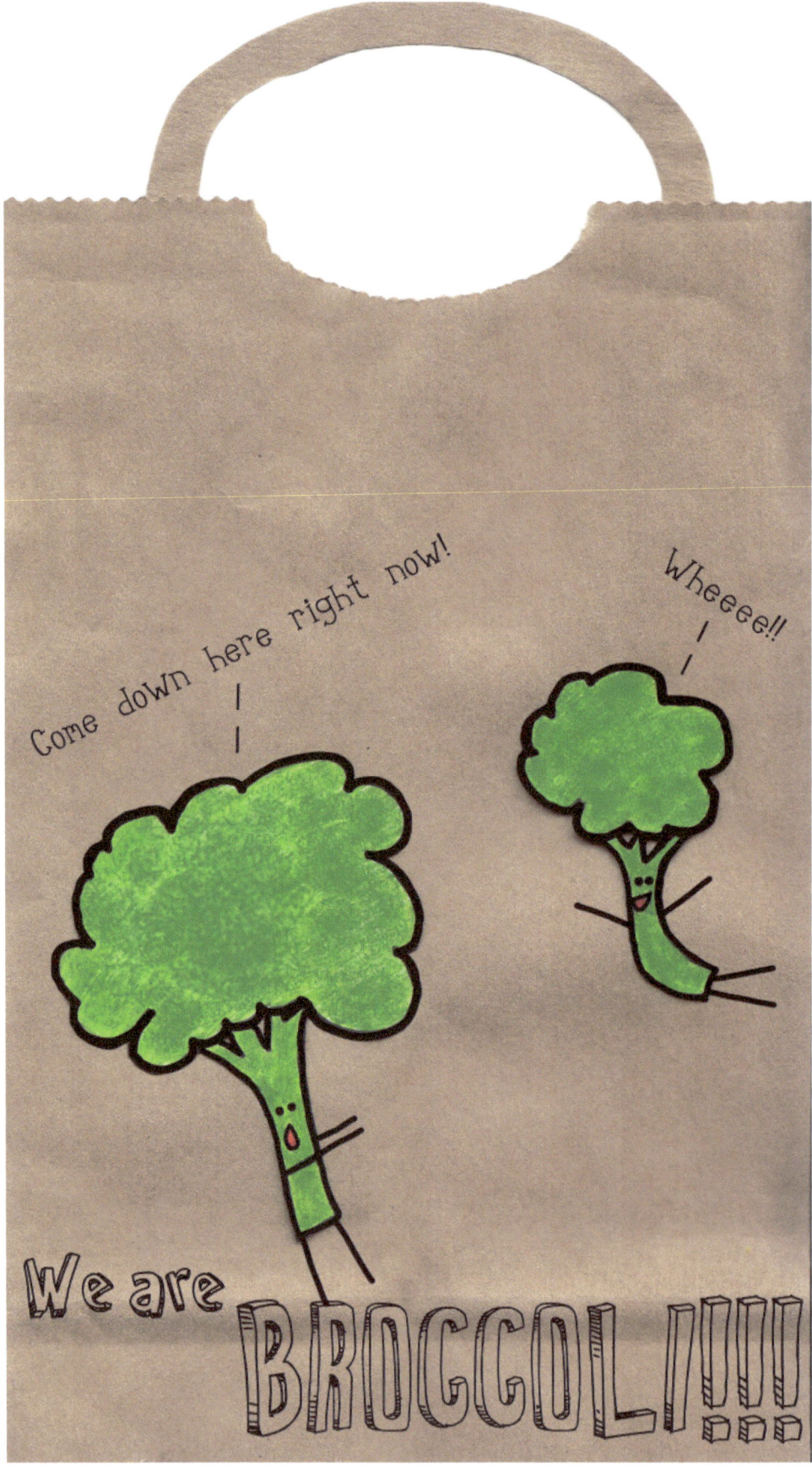

We like to have a good time, but because we're tasty, green broccoli, we also have a very serious job to do!

We rid your body of toxins, keep your lungs healthy and we are filled with all kinds of really great vitamins and nutrients that are helpful in keeping your body working at its very best!

Yummy tip:
Broccoli is great to eat raw! Cut up a head of broccoli and serve with hummus as a dip. Tell your child to pretend they're a big dinosaur and they need to eat all the trees! Whatever works, right?!

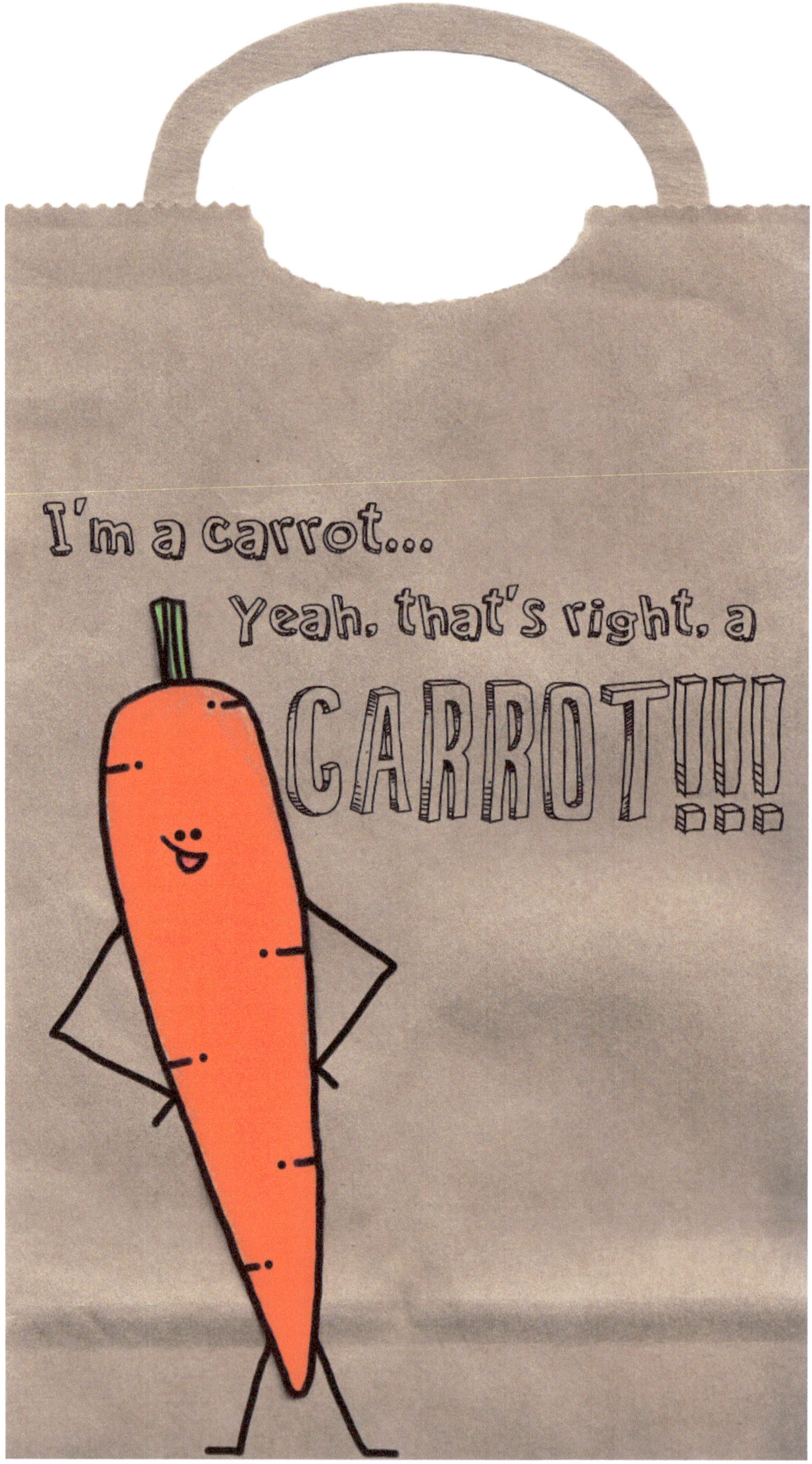
I'm a carrot...
Yeah, that's right, a
CARROT!!!

I'm orange, tasty, crunchy, and I will improve your eyesight!

I don't stop there; I also protect your heart, teeth, and gums – plus, I give your skin a beautiful glow! You're welcome!

That is something to cheer about!

Now hurry up and go eat a carrot today!

Yummy tip:

Carrots are just as good raw as they are cooked! Slice a carrot into sticks and serve with hummus as a dip – or just eat them plain! Yum!

Are you ready for us?

We're good at all kinds of stuff!

We are

CAULIFLOWER!!!

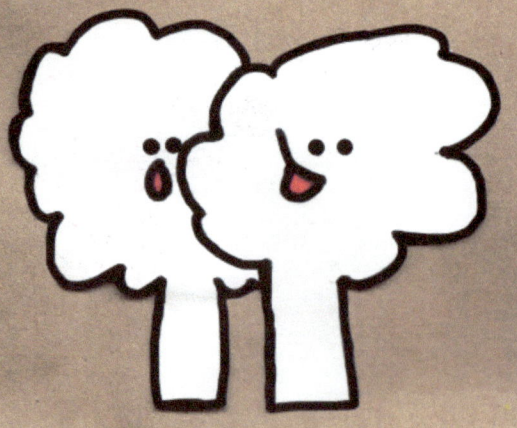

Cauliflower! How cool are we? We look like white broccoli and prevent heart disease!

We also keep your tummy as healthy as can be! Wheee!

Yummy tip:
Steam a trimmed head of cauliflower until thoroughly cooked, then mash with some butter, milk, salt and pepper - just like you're making mashed potatoes. You'll be surprised, they taste just like them!

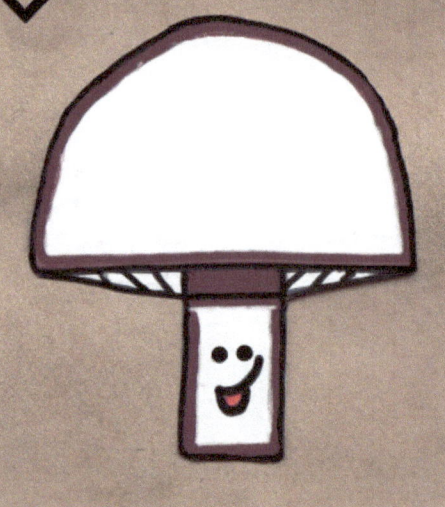

You could put mushrooms into almost any meal and our flavor is guaranteed to make you a happy kiddo!

I'm high in fiber, protein *and* I'm a natural antibiotic!

Some might say I'm kind of like a superhero!

Yummy tip:
Quesadillas are a great way to add in mushrooms to your child's diet. Grab a whole wheat tortilla; add some thinly sliced white mushrooms and your favorite cheese. Fold that sucker in half and grill your quesadilla on both sides until the cheese is melted! Top with some fresh salsa for a great tasting and quick treat!

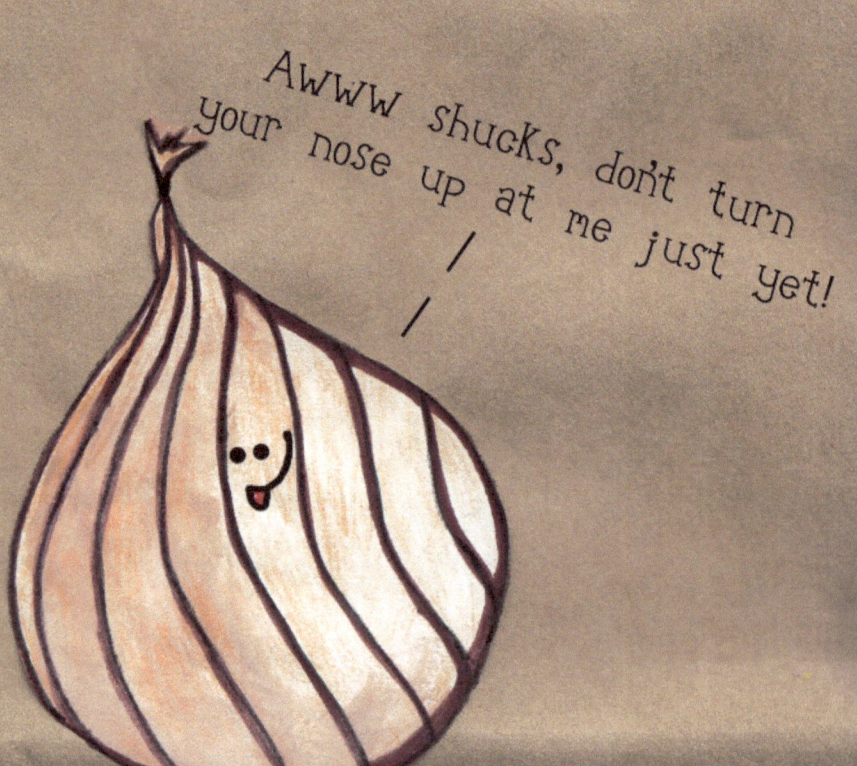

Sorry if I've made you cry before, but my strong smell is just part of my charm! We onions contain super strong antioxidants that work as medicine for your body!

I can fight off things like allergies and asthma – I also provide your body calcium, which gives your bones a major boost!

I have a great, sweet flavor and believe it or not, I'm probably already in most of your favorite dishes!

Yummy tip:
Onions are tough for snacks, but luckily you can mince up some onions and add them to soup, chili, rice or pasta dishes. They get sweet and less potent tasting as you cook them longer, so slip them into as many dishes as you can!

# We are PEAS!!!

We're teeny tiny...   ...and look just like a ball!

Peas taste so sweet, and we pop in your mouth, making us fun to eat!

We may be small, but our benefits are mighty! We contain a lot of Vitamin A - and that helps your skin stay healthy and eyes stay sharp!

Roll on down our aisle next time you're at the grocery store and take us home to have a ball!

Yummy tip:
Add a cup of fresh or frozen peas to your next snack of macaroni and cheese.

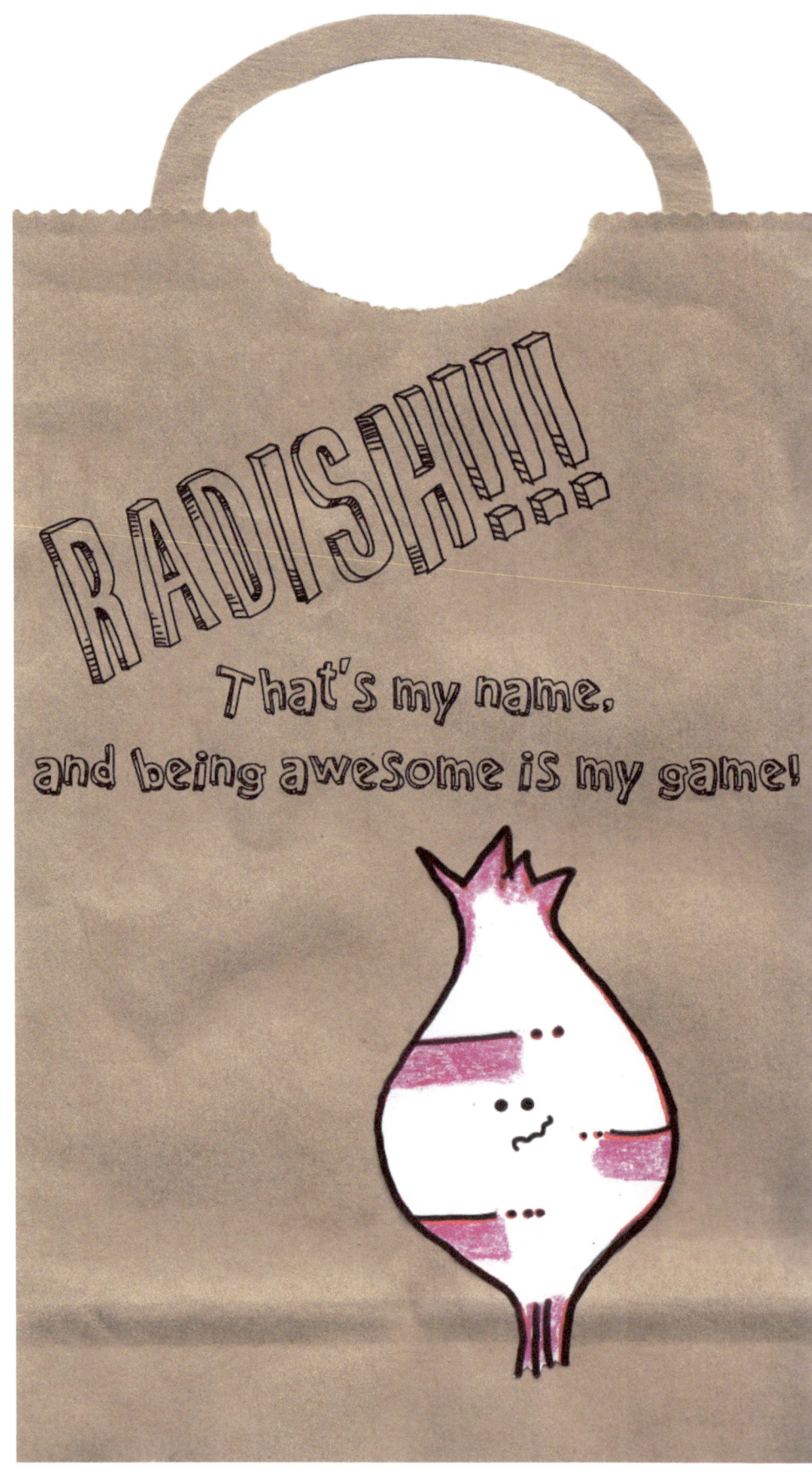

Zip-zippy-doo!

I have a bite to me, but don't worry; I don't bite! Speaking of bite, radishes work hard to keep your teeth healthy!

I also contain a healthy dose of fiber, which can help your tummy feel better!

Yummy tip:
Thinly slice radishes and add them to salads or a stir-fry. They brighten up any dish and make them look more exciting!

I'm sure you know who we are...
everyone does; we are very popular.

Yep, we're...

# STRAWBERRIES!!!

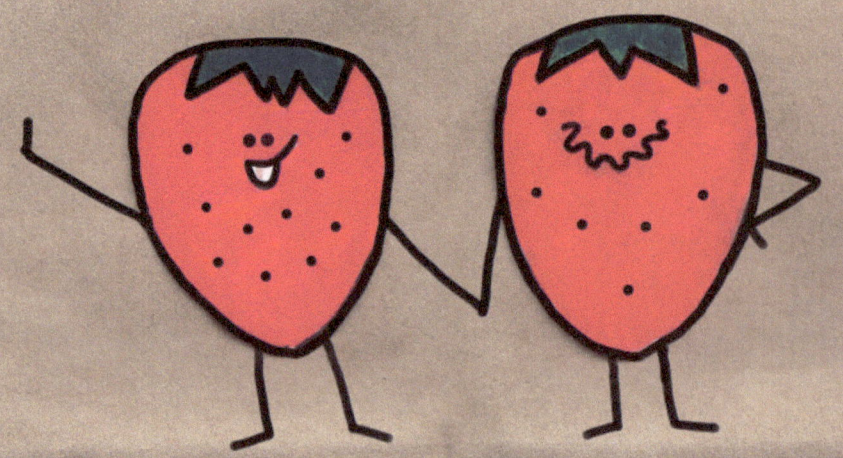

We are sweet, juicy and fun to eat, but guess what? Strawberries also help your body maintain a healthy blood pressure, keep you safe from chronic illness and are a great source of fiber.

We are a real treat for your taste buds <u>and</u> your body!

Yummy tip:
Do strawberries really need any help? While they are wonderful on their own, they are also great as an add-in. For example, add a cup of strawberries to a smoothie.  For an easy dessert, simply top sliced strawberries with whipped cream. For a quick lunch, spread a medium whole wheat tortilla with natural peanut butter and top with sliced strawberries, bananas, blueberries and then roll it all up!

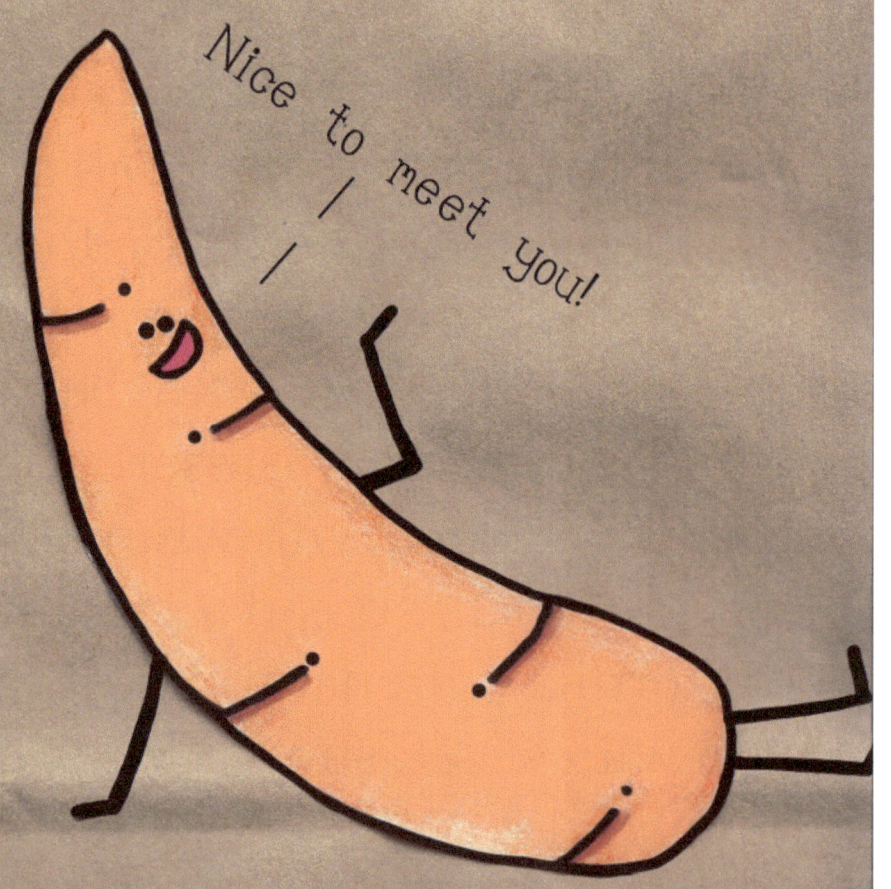

Rich and sugary, sweet potatoes are some of the tastiest things around!

I'm full of vitamin B-6! Eat some of me and your heart, nerves, skin, bones and mood will jump for joy! I'm not just for Thanksgiving dinner, so give thanks for having such a tasty treat!

Yummy tip:
Bake a sweet potato the same way you would bake a potato, 375 degrees for about 35 minutes (oven times will vary). Mash, and then add some butter, cinnamon and a touch of brown sugar. Delicious, easy and sweet!

Ketchup, tomato soup, pizza sauce - I make all of those!

Yep, I'm a...

# TOMATO!!!

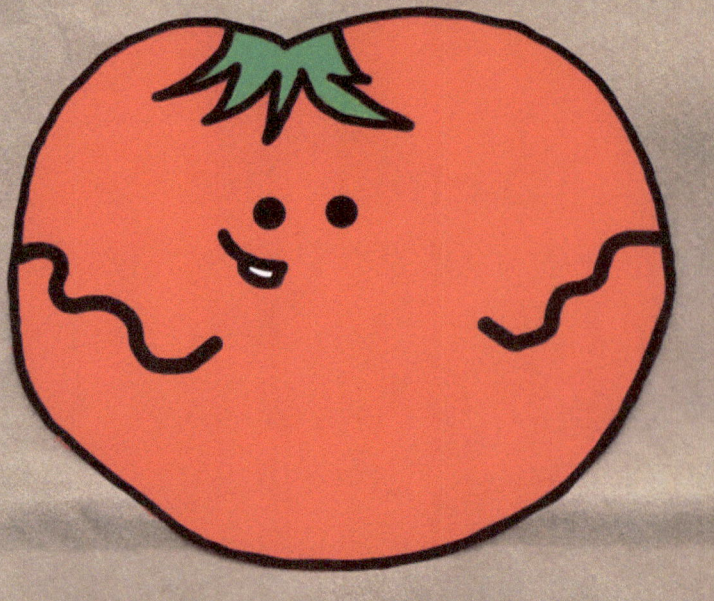

Guess what? While you're enjoying my amazing tomato taste, I'm fighting illnesses, preventing cancer and keeping you at a healthy weight! I'm also an excellent source of Vitamin C!

Whew, I gotta go - I have a lot of work to do!

Yummy tip:
Slice up a ripe tomato, some fresh mozzarella and a few fresh basil leaves. Drizzle with olive oil and sprinkle with salt and pepper. Voila, you now have the perfect salad to get the kiddos used to enjoying tomatoes.

So, kids - eat your veggie wedgies and your fruity tooties, because life is so much better when you have a healthy body!

Before we go, we just want to say:

Eat local and organic when you can!

How can you do this? Well, here are a few ways:

- Go to farmer's markets when possible. Usually May through October.
- Grow a vegetable garden
- Shop at grocery stores that support local farmers and have organic options.

# About the Author

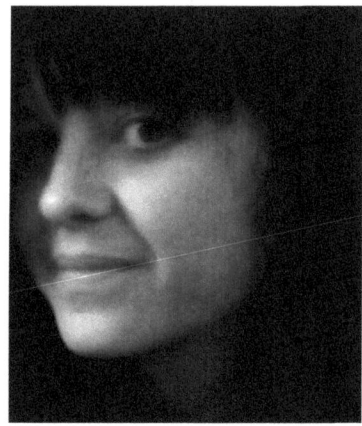

Allison Ria Duran is a mother of two and an organic/natural food enthusiast. Cooking, writing, sewing and spending time with her family are a few of her favorite things. Allison lives in Kansas City.

www.ingramcontent.com/pod-product-compliance
Lightning Source LLC
Chambersburg PA
CBHW060839290526
45792CB00006BB/1984